So
You Can Hear
the Butterfly's Song

Carol Jones Ph.D.

outskirts
press

This book is dedicated to Steve, who
always cleans up after I'm through.

TABLE OF CONTENTS

Introduction

I've always been attracted to butterflies. Just as birds represent the soul, butterflies are mythologically and historically associated with transformation.

You may have heard as a child that a butterfly landing on you was a portentous event that would bring good fortune. As a symbol of metamorphosis throughout the ages, butterflies have spiritual significance.

In the 1960s, according to chaos theory, the question became could a little butterfly, a liminal thing really, existing on the edge of nonexistence have a major impact on the world?

The theory became known as the butterfly effect. Hmm? I wonder.

Right now, we face a conundrum. Our present time is difficult, unprecedented really, but life will unfold as it will. The universe watches with patience as we make our way into the unknown.

Our lives are guided by rhythms that can't be altered by will alone. Life is a journey of events, changes we experience. Things arise and disappear.

In order to make our way into the undiscovered future, we must break from our personal chrysalis and become fully present to the transformation and to the meaning. Our present circumstances are indeed frightening, challenging, and uncomfortable, but nevertheless life will go on as we struggle to find a new path. We learn lessons during times when we are desolate that can't be learned at any other time.

The present pandemic has taught us patience and that we must find joy in the present moment. Patience and openness can allow us to watch ourselves learning and growing and becoming stronger. This time can be used for personal metamorphosis and transformation.

A collection of reflections and meditations designed to tickle you into considering alternative ways of looking at your life, *You Can Sometimes Hear the Butterfly's Song* invites you to find more meaning and purpose in your life. That's what this book is all about.

Sometimes You Can Hear the Butterfly's Song

Musing and Meditations for the New Time

I CAN ALMOST feel the itchy-tickle again as I did as a little child, lying in the grass in the backyard under the big old jacaranda tree that I liked to climb. There were dandelions to blow on then as well, before Marathon grass seed.

Pixie, my little black cocker, was usually somewhere around, yapping at the birds and foraging for the green fruits that had dropped from the gnarly old guava tree. I don't think she liked them; they were just something to smell and claim custody of after the birds had been picking at them.

I could barely sense the good, fresh, bleachy aroma of the spanking-clean sheets my nana had hung on the line in the warm, breezy air. I remember watching the butterflies, many of them monarchs, flittering above me. (It seems like there were more of them then, doesn't it?)

As I watched those butterflies, existing on the edge of nothingness in the what-if place, they were glittering things. They floated along with such delicacy that it seemed as if I could hear them chatting among themselves. Occasionally, if I listened for it, I thought I could even hear them singing.

In summer, because we didn't have a pool, I played in a wading pool with my pals, or we'd run through the sprinklers. Sometimes we played tetherball or made up pretend games and became princesses or fairies or pirates. We jumped and climbed and ran through hidden spaces and green thickets guided by our guardian angels, melting marginal monsters with our magic wands—poof!

The butterflies might dance above us like ephemeral, delicate fluttering gemstones, but they didn't sing. Butterflies seemed magical. After all, they go through four stages of life. They undergo holometabolism—presto chango, a complete change in body form.

Only when I was alone and there was some quiet could I hear them in song.

When you're little, you don't know some things are impossible, so you experiment. You no doubt think many things are within the limits of possibility; Santa Claus, Peter Pan, and the Tooth Fairy could all be real. Why not? Before you became self-aware, if you grew up in a reasonable family with no neglect or abuse, problems with self-esteem and self-efficacy were nonexistent. The entire world sighed in its beauty, and you gloried in its freshness and in your dreams. If your childhood was a difficult one, the world still held you in its mothering embrace, and you felt that you were one with everything that is.

Only later did we become isolated by believing in our own separateness. As we grew, the world shrank and was no longer part of us. But then, as adults, there was a muffled longing, a yearning for our earlier wholeness and closeness to the natural world.

How often as grown-ups do we give ourselves a chance to explore how we're feeling about things? Usually we're encouraged to ignore them, to "get a life," to curb our self-talk, to put our heads down and work through things. But like a butterfly, we all go through stages that hopefully help us to reach as far as we can in becoming responsible, mature, fully developed, and wise human beings

Perhaps, with the new paradigm, thanks to

COVID, our focus has changed, allowing us time for reflection and musing. So, maybe that's one good thing. We have all experienced times in our lives when the pressure feels unbearable. We endure one loss and then another and another. We wonder when it will all be over and we can return to a semblance of normality. When we find ourselves facing more than we can handle, we may find that the kindest thing we can do is to love ourselves and accept that we are overwhelmed and exhausted. We can love ourselves with compassion anyway. But how do we move through any type of trauma, loss, or grief without suffering from the residual psychological ramifications?

You can create your own inner therapist! You can learn to get in touch with the part of you that is healing in and of itself, the part of you that is compassionate and forgiving. Despite everything, that aspect of you can be quite powerful and can go a long way to helping you not only heal, but also find meaning and grow.

Elizabeth Kubler-Ross, in her book *On Death and Dying*, describes the five stages of working through grief. In her model, the five stages are denial, anger, bargaining, depression, and acceptance. These emotions are not linear; they can occur in any sequence and can even bounce back and forth. A sixth necessary phase has been posited by

David Kessler, who co-wrote *Grief and Grieving* with Kubler-Ross. He continues the work in his book *Finding Meaning: The Sixth Stage of Grief* and theorizes that to gain understanding and completion, there is a need to find the meaning of what has happened in order to make some sense of the events.

Recently there has been a lot of buzz about meditation, particularly mindfulness meditation, as being beneficial to our well-being. With all that has happened, a meditative state may not seem very easy to achieve. Self-reflection is valuable in discovering and accepting what has passed. New insights are free to emerge as they will need to, as undoubtedly life in the brave new world will take on a different meaning and may move in different, unique directions.

Our destiny cannot be blocked; as the old song says, "Que será, será." But in the meantime, our present is challenging, uncomfortable, unknowable, and frightening. Nonetheless, there it is.

Our job is to focus on the simple joys of being. Allow new foci to gain ascendance and new projects will gain momentum.

Whether you search for self-realization, a reinvigorated spiritual nature, or self-actualization, reflection on life's lessons may lead you to new insights. There are lessons we learn during these serene, mindful times that may seem insignificant, yet at other times these learnings are not available to us and may become relevant when you least expect it. There are many things to learn in this "between" time.

The growing body of information on the mind-body connection suggests that by focusing your attention on meditation and mindfulness exercises you can profoundly enhance your relaxation response. The relaxation response helps to reduce blood lactate, that nasty little critter partially responsible for stress headaches. It also helps improve the immune system, enhances metabolism, and improves brain function and attention. When you're relaxed, you feel more connected to others, and in this time of isolation that's a good thing. It also increases serotonin (the feel-good hormone) and improves mood and energy.

Spiritual healers, shamans, and psychologists have long sought to examine the advantages of accessing the inner child, the one without limits or boundaries, the playful child who is connected with nature. This child-self can be transformative.

Creativity, adaptability, and resilience are the hallmarks of this inner child. New strategies for coping with life can be the end result.

Give yourself permission to dance to your own rhythms. Let your heart open to the simple things that make you happy. Discover your artistry, and enlarge your capacity to become more caring and creative in your life. Explore all it means to be you. Speculate that new possibilities may yet be available. It's time to learn more empathy, sympathy, and compassion for yourself and for others.

Sitting with legs crossed may not be for everyone, but mindfulness requires nothing more than clearing one's mind and focusing, outwardly or inwardly. It's like taking a little vacation from the clutter of your self-speak.

Using the following guided imagery exercises and brief meditations will enhance your ability to muse and become more mindful, to relax and use your imagination, and to ultimately find new perspectives and meaning.

With luck, there still remains an echo of our mutuality with the world. We may now begin to feel a part of the blessed, sacred earth. We may now be called home again.

The Time in Between

IT SOMETIMES FEELS like we are living in a time between two eras.

We haven't quite left the world of the past with its institutionalized, industrial, centrally and economically self-contained institutions. We're in a nowhere place; we haven't quite made it to the future paradigm. This can be a dangerous time. The fate of the planet may rest in the balance. We cling to the past because we haven't quite grasped what the new worldview will be. It's our responsibility. It all depends on the choices we make. Awareness of these choices helps us to access more realistically how our decisions affect others. We cannot solve the problems we have collectively created with the same type of thinking that created them. Yet, sadly, at this point some things may really be out of our hands. Frightening!

How do we embrace this uncertainty and glean from it new opportunities? How can we perceive even a glimmer of the new road ahead through the dark woods of conflicting ideas, confusion, and doubt?

This present-future time is new territory. The world has changed so much, so quickly. We are forced to contemplate a landscape beyond the scope of our experience. What course will the future take? Shall there be continued overpopulation and a proliferation of new pandemics or other nuclear or chemical catastrophes? Or, will we find ways to sustain ourselves and the earth's resources at the same time? Will original thinking and telecommunication contribute to true planetary integration with an emphasis on social justice and understanding our connection to one another?

Crisis can give rise to quantum shifts and creative adaptations.

Shall our world be a place that adapts and develops solutions? Will we transform the structure of society? Will all people be given a chance to develop their potential to grow and to find meaning in their lives? What will we learn from the past? There is such a sense of ambiguity that we feel paralyzed to choose.

But choose we must. In this challenge there is also some allure. The possibilities of the future beckon us, inviting us to explore them. The mystery evokes our curiosity. We must, therefore, approach it carefully and thoughtfully.

NATURE

WHEN ALL OF our attention is only directed to how wrong things are, we're hobbled and lose our power to act effectively.

But nature offers us a panacea. Nature makes no judgments and provides us with a glimpse of infinity. Natural, wild places can draw us to experience vitality. Wild places quietly remind us that we are uniquely ourselves. With so much of the human experience now removed from nature, we forget that we are a part of it. A bevy of studies have added to the growing literature on the benefits of spending time in the outdoors.

As we grow up and months and years go by, we discover and explore all the sights and sounds and gizmos of the virtual and synthetic world. That world can be intriguing and amazing, but the longing for nature and its gifts remains.

If we allow ourselves to listen, nature clambers, nearly harangues us to allow it in, demanding that we feel its force and its dazzling dynamic aliveness. It's hard to know just what it is about nature that makes us feel better even when we are down. Do certain colors or shapes trigger neurochemicals in our visual cortex? Or is it just that people who live close to park-like places get more exercise and therefore more oxygen to their brains? It's been found that even looking at pictures of the great outdoors can calm people and sharpen their performance—simply looking, nothing more, without judgment or expectations.

If they look for a long enough period of time, people feel a sense of joy. This is an example of a simple meditation.

Nature urges us to feel its watery surges and to be impaled by its passionately pungent greens and yellows and blues and crimsons. It challenges us to feel deliciously loamy. It defies us to ignore its cracked, rock-hard cold shell and its bewildering assortment of evocative aromas.

Nature reminds us we are all implicated in each other's well-being and with nature itself. We are related to the grass and the sea. Our cells and atoms belong to the stars. When we lose our continuity with the ferns and the flowers and the worms, we may well block our connection to the life force and its power.

Studies have shown that the earth's electromagnetic field, kind of like its heartbeat, vibrates at 7.83 Hz. This discovery is known as the Schumann resonance. This field is created by thunderstorms and lightning flashes. It so happens that human brain waves, alpha waves that is, vibrate around the same frequency. We are designed to be in harmony with the earth. When we are, we're healthy. When we're not, we can exhibit signs that range from insomnia, headaches, palpitations, and anxiety to actual illness. Studies say morbid rumination (brooding) can lead to depression.

Earth's current is direct current (DC), not alternating current. Humans evolved in an environment devoid of AC magnetic fields. Unfortunately, with so many technological devices, such as computers, cell phones, and TVs, that emit electromagnetic fields that are not congruent with 7.83 Hz, we are overrun by "bad vibrations" that interfere with us being in tune with our planet.

Synthetic drugs, processed foods, and stress also can have the impact of lowering our personal frequency.

One of the best ways to improve being in harmony with the earth is the simple act of spending time in nature. It's been found that happy people really do emit good vibrations!

By joining with nature, our lives are freed to

focus on the greater pattern of which we all are a part. Once any unnatural barriers we have erected are transcended, we are free to become conduits for the natural vitality of the world.

Take a forest bath, go barefoot, build a sand castle, dig in the garden, or lie on the grass under a tree and experience those good vibrations!

FLOWER POWER—
JUST FOR FUN

For centuries mankind has attributed symbolic meanings to plants. Trees, herbs, and flowers provided man with a context for understanding the natural world, a world upon which people relied to provide them with what they needed to exist.

For Romans, wreaths of bay leaves signified peace and triumph. The Greeks felt bay was useful as a protection from witchcraft. The Chumash Indians of the California coast used bay leaves as a palliative for headaches. Those are just a few examples.

As you travel through your surroundings, notice the local flora and take a moment to think about its symbolism.

Azalea	temperance
Buttercup	humility
Camellia	good luck
Carnation	impulse
Daffodil	unrequited love
Daisy	innocence
Fuchsia	confiding love
Gardenia	purity
Gladiolus	love at first sight
Marigold	passion and creativity
Morning Glory	affection
Orchid	love and refinement
Pansy	merriment
Petunia	your presence soothes me
Poppy	magic, sleep, and rest
Rose	passion and love
Snap Dragon	strength
Sunflower	adoration

Anxious Moments
(A Meditation)

- Anxiety: a feeling of worry, nervousness, or unease, typically about an imminent event or something with an uncertain outcome.
- Synonyms: worry, concern, apprehension, consternation, foreboding, tension, stress, the shakes, the jumps, collywobbles, jim-jams.
- Symptoms:
  - » Behavioral: hypervigilance, irritability, or restlessness
  - » Cognitive: lack of concentration, racing thoughts, unwanted thoughts
  - » Whole body: fatigue or sweating
- Also common: rumination, excessive worry, fear, and feelings of impending

doom, insomnia, nausea, palpitations, or trembling.

You can start by taking about ten minutes to describe what your anxiety feels like, how it manifests. Notice what it's telling you.

What part(s) of your body let you know you're anxious? Does your heart beat faster? Do your hands get clammy? Do you feel jittery or distracted? Or do you get crabby or irritated with other people?

Were you anxious when you were little? If you were, how did your family handle your anxiety when you were a kid? Were they sympathetic or did they shine it on? In what ways is your anxiety now the same or different from the anxiety you felt when you were a child?

What is your first memory of what is presently causing your anxiety? Was it threatening physically, or did it threaten your loved ones or maybe your self-esteem?

If you get a chance during the day, take a quick note when you notice you're anxious. What event or thought provoked it?

Become compassionate with yourself when you're experiencing anxiety. Getting frustrated or angry at your "stupid" anxiety does no good. Allow yourself to show a little love and understanding toward yourself. When you've been trained to "suck up" your negative feelings, it can be pretty hard to reframe that learning and treat yourself with any kind of understanding.

Dedicate some time every day to finding a place of stillness. Remind yourself to find brief moments to enter into mindfulness.

Pema Chödrön, an American Buddhist nun, teaches Tonglen (check out her website for more information on this technique). Very simply, she suggests breathing in and out, taking the pain of anxiety in and breathing out relief and spaciousness. Of course, this seems counterintuitive to go against what we typically do with our painful feelings. (Tonglen embraces them, rather than trying to push them aside.)

Practiced over time, our mind retrains itself to accept negative feelings without fear.

The second step in this practice is to breathe in the sadness and heartbreak humanity feels in this moment—the fear, the loneliness, and the disappointment—and to breathe out your care and love.

When you can send your concern and understanding to others, you may find that your anxiety quiets itself. Remember that in some mysterious way all of us are part of the invisible web of life and are together in our feelings of pain and worry.

Conscious Living

EACH OF US arrives in the world a helpless little bundle convinced that the world exists to take care of all our wants and needs.

The egocentric toddler learns to say "mine" and "me." And of course, toddlers learn to say "no" with great alacrity! It takes a while for them to learn that the world does not revolve solely around them.

Eventually they learn to relate to and get along with others. Still, the internal petty little tyrant still wants attention.

An adult human is comprised of a complex of inner forces, including messages sent from the pesky ego-driven child who cries for comfort, hugs, and praise, and develops a myriad of self-defense mechanisms.

When the ego is left on its own to dominate the adult personality, problems arise. It is still a necessary part of the personality but must be mediated by the id and superego, the two other members of the personality triad.

If all the personality's components are modulated, the adult can go on to develop the "I" in relation to others. We become most human when we meet the other heart to heart, the "I" to "thou."

The way we talk, the way we live, and the way we behave send out ripples. We may never really know what the consequent outcomes will be. When we live in a more conscious and measured way, respecting one another, we can change the world.

When we really begin to understand that the smallest smile may help to save a life or that a miniscule meanness can break a heart or cause lasting harm, we become more measured in our behaviors, certainly.

And, in opening our hearts to life and to others, we can begin to let go of some of our fear-based defenses, and in doing so, we can help to lift the burden of our own fears.

When we awaken from the delusion of our separateness, we can become part of a greater life. We are all inextricably interrelated to each other and to all of life!

Presence

How do we get out of life's fast lane? This unusual time may offer us an answer. To enter mindfulness, we must enter the present moment. Taking things slowly may feel uncomfortable and disconcerting. We, after all, are used to moving at breakneck speeds, but with what objective in mind? Altering one's pace may put you on a path to presence.

How often do our habitual thoughts yammer at us? We are automatically conditioned by our upbringing to try to be right, to "do it right!" We have learned that it's awful if we are wrong. These ideas put a burden of pressure on us. How can we really know what's right without a context? Not everything is black or white. When you free yourself from pressure and judgment, life feels new.

"Out beyond wrongdoing and right-doing there is a field," said the thirteenth-century poet

Rumi. "I'll meet you there." That's the place to look for—where presence can be practiced.

One needs to consider two ideas: First, presence is a state that must be practiced; it does not come naturally for most people. Instinctually we are wired to watch out for our safety, and that requires that we pay attention to the nuances of our environment. Secondly, although it is hard to believe, our lives need not rely on our current mechanized society.

THE WOLVES

AN OLD CHEROKEE brave was teaching his young grandson about the ways of life.

"A fight is going on inside me," he told the boy. "Two wolves are fighting; it is a terrible fight."

"One wolf," he said, "is evil. He is anger and envy, sorrow, regret, greed, arrogance, self- pity, guilt, resentment, inferiority, lies, false pride, superiority, and ego."

He continued to tell the boy, "The other wolf is good. He is peace, joy, love, serenity, humility, kindness, benevolence, empathy, generosity, truth, compassion, and faith."

He tells his grandson that the same fight is going on inside of him and everyone else as well.

The boy considers all of his grandfather's words, and then he asks his grandfather, "Which wolf will win?"

The old Cherokee simply replied, "The one you feed."

Mindfulness (A Meditation)

Mindfulness is a form of meditation that doesn't ask you to clear your mind; in fact, it asks just the opposite. It asks that you pay attention! It focuses on becoming totally into the here and now.

Of course, this also means that you're not worrying about the future or fretting over the past. It entails noticing everything that's happening around you—what you see, what you hear, and how things smell and taste.

Give it a try.

Select a daily activity that you do when you are alone; it can pretty much be anything you like. It can be taking a walk (going for a jog probably won't work too well). It could be brushing your hair, ironing, cooking dinner, or something like that. Once you have made up your mind about the activity, practice becoming mindful by noticing every thought and sensation that comes to your consciousness and what it evokes for you.

Let's start with trying it in the shower.

In the shower, for example, you may notice the soap and the way it slips over your skin. How does it feel? If you sniff it, what kind of aroma do you perceive? Is it flowery, astringent, or woody, or maybe it smells like fresh laundry? What comes to mind for you?

What color is the shower? Is the water hot and steamy or rather cool and invigorating or somewhere in between? If you're shampooing, what does the shampoo smell like? What does it remind you of?

You'll probably notice how the drops of water cling to the curtain or the shower door and then run like tears or little streams down to the floor.

Is the floor made of a fiberglass shower pan or is it tiled? Is there a shower mat? Does it feel a little slippery or does it feel secure?

And if you're using a washcloth, take note of its condition. Is it a little old and rough, or is it soft and new?

You get the idea. This type of meditation requires that you be in the present and gives you a little vacation from overthinking things.

The Life Path

IT'S ONLY WHEN the path vanishes that we become aware it's no longer beneath our feet. Everything feels all wrong. In a panic we try to retrace our steps. Either we rediscover the path and resume our way along it, maybe in some small way transformed, or we stumble disconcertedly until we find ourselves upon a new one, grateful for some sense of familiarity in the feel of it under our feet, although now unsure of our destination.

We search for a path through life that we can call our own. Our chosen life path serves as a cipher for the purpose and meaning we have in life. It stands as a kind of banner that decries what we value and hope for. It allows us to believe in the fantasy that we are purposeful and know what lies ahead. The path feels safe; it allows us to move freely with some assurance that we know where we are and where we are going.

We worry that if we lose the path, we'll ramble aimlessly, depressed or despairing. To lose one's path forces thought, effort, and a requirement to take pause to consider and overcome unexpected barriers. We can become paralyzed by the anxiety and obsessed by our fearful predicament, as we are forced to negotiate metaphysical rocks, crevasses, and uprooted trees.

We do have a choice though. We can emerge from the morass by accepting that we lack an obvious path to follow. We can become free to respond spontaneously, liberated to find our way over perceived barriers as we reframe them as possible vehicles for new discoveries.

Perhaps we must learn not to react from fixed perspectives, but to take a dynamic motile position as we learn to create abundance from our discoveries.

The Real World

WHAT DO YOU suppose are the parameters of reality? If you ascribe to the belief that there are infinite realities, then at some level everything you experience is in some sense real. But then, the things you have not yet experienced are part of reality as well. Since your experiences make up such a small and unique range of possibilities within this infinity, they constitute only an inkling of reality.

Like an archaic map colorfully embellished with implausible and fantastical creatures, your experiences are a simile for a whole range of potential realities meant to be discovered and explored.

It seems that what we now know may be valid as far as it goes, but it cannot possibly be representative of the whole of things. The world is no longer believed to be flat. Nevertheless, we all live in our own independent psychic universes. We tentatively agree on somewhat fuzzy concepts that we have embraced and that have been dictated through our language and cultural mores, beliefs that are the consensus of our time.

But there is one of Buddha's teachings that speaks of two truths. First, there is absolute truth. It points to ultimate reality, that we are all made of energy, and stardust, atoms, and particles of light. On this level there is only oneness, but we need to honor the second truth, relative truth, as well. It's a place where our actions count and the relationship between cause and effect matters.

So, the old perspective will simply not do for the future. If we ignore the relative reality and just live in the absolute dimension, we aren't experiencing the whole of life. But stepping out of our comfort zone takes courage and may ultimately change our beliefs about reality.

Two thousand years ago, Plato explored the problem of a limited perspective of reality in his allegory of the cave. He asks us to imagine that in a cave was a group of prisoners, shackled from childhood, who could only see in front of them. These people could only see shadows projected on a blank wall. The sounds of people talking (those who imprisoned them) echoed off the wall, and the prisoners believed that the muffled, echoey words came from the shadows. For them, these shadows seemed real. After all, they were all the prisoners had ever known: the shadows shaped their reality.

Eventually, one of the prisoners escaped the cave and was confronted with the bright sunshine and the colors and textures of the world, that is to say, the truth of things. If he returned to the cave, he knew he wouldn't be believed! He'd be laughed at. But his version of reality had changed forever.

Plato's allegory explores the tension of perceived reality (the shadows) versus the reality that is the truth.

So, there may be more to it than we think. Believing that we know the whole truth may keep us from learning an important lesson. Being aware of this blind spot frees us to grow in understanding.

Who knows?

Imagine
(Guided Imagery)

IMAGINE ITS MIDMORNING on a late spring day. Imagine you're lying on an old, striped beach towel in a field of spring grasses; some seem very green, some seem almost chartreuse. The contrast is lovely.

You used a few of the willowy, yellow-flowered weeds to dare your friends to eat when you were a kid. What were they called anyway, something like oxalis maybe? Yeah, that was it. You decide to try one now. "Hmm," you think, "not bad really, interesting taste."

On the edge of the field is a thicket—almost a woodland—of gnarly old oak trees. Their mismatched limbs like a tangle of yarn allow beams of sunshine to make surreal shadows on the leaf-littered ground.

As you relax with your head on your faded, much-used backpack, you regard the cumulus clouds like white pillows, skittering in the true-blue sky above you. There must be some turbulence up there, you decide, as they are moving quickly. The feeling is one of relaxation.

Out of the corner of your eye you see an older man moving out from the oaks. He's wearing unusual clothes, dun colored, almost like a monk or an actor in an old biblical movie. It's a long, belted robe of some type.

"That's strange," you think.

You're not frightened, just interested. His appearance is not threatening but quite peaceful. As he moves closer, you remain supine. He approaches and introduces himself. His voice is melodious, singsong, almost hypnotizing. He tells you he has something he wants you to know.

He folds himself down to sit on the grass next to you. He sighs and begins to speak. He delivers his message. He rises and turns and begins to walk back into the trees.

You consider what he has told you. Feeling quite sleepy, you close your eyes and fall into a dreamy sleep.

When you awaken, you feel serene and very satisfied.

A One-Way Street

HOW CAN WE wean ourselves from thinking that life is a one-way street? We miss a lot by not allowing ourselves to consider multiple possibilities. When we look at things from one point of view, we miss nuance and complexity and potentiality.

Like the African tribespeople who don't even recognize themselves in snapshots or mirrors, when we isolate ourselves in a personal perspective and disallow dialogue with others, we live in fear, in passive uninvolvement and can't see the flowing textures of life that surround us. We lose our freshness and vivid spontaneity.

Although some of the messages that the world is sending us may feel cryptic and despairing and can only be understood over time, at least when you stay in the present and open to undertones, you can choose from vast, multidimensional options.

From these options we can choose to make decisions, take risks, gain new perspectives, and live more fully.

Rush

WHERE DOES THE time go? There never seems to be enough of it. We don't have enough of it for ourselves, nor do we have time for each other. Most of us are scheduled months in advance and feel guilty about wasting time.

We are always on the way to something, never being anywhere. The faster we go, the more gizmos we buy to act as surrogate secretaries and babysitters, which are themselves a waste our time with all the programming they require. Smartphones have made us always accessible. They exhort us with their nagging tenacity to be on time for appointments and remind us of everything else.

We certainly are well organized but also less spontaneous. How can we consider even thinking about enjoying the present when failing in the future is in the back of our minds like Stephen King's

Langoliers chomping their way relentlessly at our backs, urging us to hurry up?

It's all about getting as many things done as quickly as possible—fast lane, fast food, fast sex. Our to-do list looks more like an airplane schedule. When will I have time to exercise, to meditate, or to read? When can I squeeze in playing with the kids or calling my friends? Days are so full there's no room to breathe.

Now that it's all been overturned, a new paradigm can develop.

COVID has given us the time to find a quiet peaceful spot, a place where we can pause and listen and reflect on what our hearts and bodies and the world around us have to say.

Stay encouraged that you will find that place.

WILD JOURNEY

HAVE YOU EVER found yourself in a place that just doesn't feel right? Do you ever feel that, despite trying to play the game according to the rules, you don't quite know why you're here or what it is you're doing—or even why you're trying to do it? Perhaps you tried to make some positive changes and those changes have made you feel more out of sync with everything. Maybe you've been looking back on your life and thinking that you had it pretty good. Now you're wondering why you bothered to rock the boat in the first place. Such issues have compelled and confounded theologians and philosophers for centuries.

So what if you *do* feel lost? At least you've taken some risks. And if you've lost your way, you must have had *some* destination in mind.

Perhaps you're just afraid to wonder, "What

will I find? Is this really what's right for me?" Or, you may be thinking, "In what ways will I change? Who will I become?"

How you take the first step, through your heart or your head, intentionally or inadvertently, is entirely up to you. The one thing you can be certain of is that things will not be predictable.

When you travel in new territory, there's an almost irresistible urge to smooth over the strangeness, to make it like something you know, though in doing so you miss the uniqueness of the place. It's bound to be a bewildering experience.

The journey can be awkward and perilous. You don't, after all, know exactly what you're searching for. There is a loss of moorings as the old self slips away. What replaces your former certitude are confusion and vulnerability and openness and ultimately something new.

Remember, no matter how lost you feel, there will come a time when you feel right at home again.

LETTING BEAUTY IN
(A MEDITATION)

FIND A QUIET place in a natural setting, if possible. If that isn't possible, find a place that has some interesting things to regard. Make yourself comfortable in a relaxed sitting position. As you settle in, become aware of your breathing. Remember to focus on your diaphragm and notice your breath moving in and out slowly and evenly.

Look at your surroundings. Are your sensory experiences interesting in any way? Do you smell any unusual odors? What about the light—is it bright, cloudy, vibrant, or subdued? And is the temperature warmish or cool?

And what about you? Are you feeling anxious or bored, or maybe comfortable and relaxed?

As your awareness opens, you might notice a

quality that is different, a quality that reveals itself when awareness and form come together and enfold into one another.

As you open up the book of the world, it unfolds before you and inside you. Like a scholar of renown, you begin to discern more subtlety, with more depth, and finally, with more beauty. The beauty whispers to you in some undefinable way, urging you to unite with it, to pass into it, to let the beauty wash over you and become part of you.

This beauty, what many call God, coexists with the presence. It does not reveal itself, except by the instrument of attention to it and your willingness to receive it.

Due to some judgment, some lack of attention, how often do we shut out beauty rather than take it in? Beauty reveals itself solely to the extent that we are open to it.

To be open to the moment brings it and us to life. When we lack presence, we're just going through the motions. We're faking it—unaware, no feeling, no color, flat.

With presence there is knowing. Without presence we are not invited to enter into this union with the beautiful.

As babies we come into this world open wide, but we learn to modulate our instinctive awareness as we grow. Finally, as adults we operate in a state where things don't fully register, and we just ride with it.

To experience beauty you must commit; you must engage it. This doesn't come naturally to most people: for many people practice at being present is critical.

You can quiet your mind, witness your thoughts, and let go of distractions.

This can bring you closer to the heart of stillness, which can help you to balance your life and to find renewal. Letting everything be, just as it is, opens you to the experience of beauty, joy, and communion.

WORRIES AND FEARS

HOW AWKWARD THAT the recent necessity for social distance has presented us with a kind of conundrum. On the one hand, it may truly be a lifesaver; on the other, social distancing flies in the face of the notion that we have just started to explore, that spiritually at any rate, we are a world community. The crisis certainly displaced the idea that many strive for: oneness with the universe.

You've probably heard it repeated over and over that we are "all in this together," and yet physically, this premise of togetherness can be quite dangerous and may be for some time.

Perhaps it's helpful to recognize the newness of the situation. We are generally a gregarious and social bunch, we humans. But we can also be adaptable and creative.

Numerous novel and impromptu ideas have

come about already. Virtual cocktail and dinner parties as well as playdates have been set up. Do these ersatz encounters fill a need? Perhaps they do, perhaps they do not.

Certainly, teleconferences have become the lifesaver for many businesses and may be adopted in the future. They offer people the option to save fuel as well as other resources, after all.

And I'm sure there are many who would just as well have a designated shopper do the work of going to the grocery store. It would free the buyers for other tasks. They might decide never go back to the old ways even when allowed!

So many worries and fears occupy our minds that we wind up going around and around with constant "what ifs?"

When one is so distracted, it's not easy to accomplish much of anything. Since we are so concerned and involved with things that are external to us and to all the mixed messages we are constantly receiving, it can really be easy to overlook what's going on inside of us.

Perhaps a good idea is to step away from all the concerns that occupy our minds and take a "time-out" to look at our inner selves. This can give the mind, the body and the spirit the time that they need to reenergize and regain vitality and to heal.

Taking a break may not seem to be very

productive, but spending a little time in nature, working on a few yoga asanas, paying attention to the breath or having a bubble bath helps us to focus on mindfulness and help us come to realize the we are not able to control much, (which was actually always true) but at least we are able to bring to all that we encounter a better, and more positive outlook.

Hopefully, this spiritual and disciplined self-distancing from our quotidian worries will lessen the weight of our contradicting and confusing thoughts and perceived troubles and will allow us to become more receptive to the wealth of wisdom the universe has to offer.

SOME PEOPLE DON'T
– SOME PEOPLE DO

How DO YOU choose what to do, or how you want to be? Certainly, its complicated. Poet Laureate Robert Frost said he took the road less traveled and that made all the difference. How do you choose which path to travel? Will you continue on a path that is somewhat consistent with the one you've been traveling on or are you able to break away and go in a different, perhaps more tangential direction?

Which choice is better, what values do you believe have more import? Which path will cost you more: which path will be of more benefit? What will the tangible gains be? How do you ever really know?

How will you change if you choose to be

different or try something new? What will you have to give up?

How willing are you to experience loss, grief, limitations and the possibility of disappointment or defeat? How might you grow from risking the changes you may make?

How will you choose?

- Some people don't want to be sick.
- Some people don't want to live in the limelight.
- Some people don't want to die
- Some people don't want to live
- Some people don't want to be cold
- Some people don't want to be afraid
- Some people don't want to be alone.
- Some people don't want to be small.
- Some people don't want to be big.
- Some people don't want to be different.
- Some people don't want to be like other people.
- Some people don't want to go to hell.
- Some people don't want to be lonely.
- Some people don't want to live by the rules.
- Some people want to talk with God.
- Some people want to be God.
- Some people want to die honorably.
- Some people want to save mankind.

- Some people want to rule the world.
- Some people want to go to heaven.
- Some people want power.
- Some people want to have a lot of money
- Some people want to have a perfect body.
- Some people want to be famous.
- Some people want to be a better person.
- Some people want to learn more.
- Some people want to be alone
- Some people want to help others.
- Some people want to make a difference.

And you?

Who Knows – (A Meditation)

Find a spot that's private and tranquil. Take a few minutes to focus and relax.

Make some room for yourself to either sit comfortably or else lie down.

As you rest quietly and breathe easily, feel yourself begin to relax. Notice the regularity of your breathing. Does your breathing take place in your chest or your abdomen? Or is it a combination of both. Place your hand on your abdomen on top of your belly button and notice if you feel your stomach moving in and out. You might like to think about waves or the wind. As you inhale will your stomach to recede, ebbing back to your spine. As you exhale allow your stomach to flow forward again. Notice how relaxed you are beginning to feel.

Notice the sounds around you. If you are outside the sounds will obviously be different than if you are inside. Do you hear cars going by, clocks ticking? Birds tweeting? Is your stomach growling? Are bees buzzing? Is an air conditioner humming? Focus your attention on these minutiae and then let them go.

Notice how relaxed you are feeling. Are you a little warm, a little cool or are you feeling just right? What time of day is it? Is it a time of day when you usually feel energized or are you a little groggy? As you consider your physical situation make note of it and then let it go and relax a little more deeply.

As you think about how you are feeling ask yourself if there are any people who have truly made an impression on you. Are there say, three people you would say have really affected you either positively or negatively. What kind of an impact did these people have on you? Did they change you in some way? Did they influence the person you are today? What exactly was it about these people who had such an impact on you? What type of power or authority did they wield? How were they connected to you?

Are they still in your life?

Has the impact they had been positive or negative? If the influence was a negative one, is it still operant in your life today? If the influence was a positive one, would you like to keep it operating in your current situation? What did you learn from each of these people? One interesting thing to think about is that taking a good look at issues like someone's negative impact may surprise you. You might discover that you may still have gotten something positive from them. You learned how you absolutely didn't want to be at any rate. You made lemonade from your lemons, became a stronger person. Certainly, that is a good thing.

And what about anybody who has been a good influence in your life? Have you incorporated this person's positive traits into your own repertoire? If not, why not?

Many people can't think of anyone that they truly admire. That's OK. If you can't think of anyone who has truly inspired you, fantasize a little about what this type of inspirational person would be like. What values would he or she cherish? How would this person have suffered in his or her life and what obstacles would this individual have overcome? How would this person have become so unique or so wise and inspirational? How would this person behave and which goals would he or she aspire to?

What would this person look like on paper? What about this person would you most admire? Is this fantasy person anything like you? How? If you had encountered this individual, what traits would you emulate and what would you learn from this person about the unique individual *you* would like to become?

Compassion –
(Guided Imagery)

Be Compassionate With Yourself

Lie or sit in a comfortable position. It's helpful to close your eyes. Notice where your body is experiencing tension. Take a few calming breaths. Check your body again for areas that are still tense. As you discover them, breathe into them.

Relax your muscles. Starting at your neck and working your way down your body. Notice as you continue to breathe how the breath affects the muscles.

You may begin to experience images, that's fine, accept what comes to you.

Now imagine that you're in a cozy quiet room with a comfortable chair facing you. Imagine that you see yourself sitting in the chair. Notice your posture. Notice your facial expression. Notice what you're wearing, you may even notice that you're dressed as you are now!

Now imagine what the image of yourself is saying to you:

> I am a worthy human being. I am a good person who exists and who is trying not only to survive, but also to grow and better myself. I take myself seriously. I take myself into consideration first in all aspects of my life. But I also consider the needs of others.
>
> I have legitimate desires and legitimate needs. I don't need to justify myself to others when I make choices. I take responsibility for the choices that I make.
>
> I try to do my best, but because I'm human, I do make mistakes. When I do make a mistake, I try to learn what I can from it. I know I am imperfect, but I try to forgive myself for my mistakes. Sometimes finding forgiveness is difficult.
>
> I am aware that others are equally as worthy I am and equally as imperfect as well. I have compassion for them because they struggle, as do I, to stay alive and get their needs met.

Imagine that the figure in the chair—that is, you—rises from the chair and comes over to the place where you are sitting. Imagine that the figure merges with you, the observer, to make one whole and complete person.

Relax and be at peace with yourself. Breathe and float, very relaxed. When you are ready, open your eyes and come back to your space and the here and now. Enjoy the feeling of the relaxation and refreshment. And notice a sense of acceptance toward yourself and others.

THE POWER OF MYTH

WHY DO YOU suppose myths are so fascinating? Author Joseph Campbell would tell us that we are drawn to mythic tales because they resonate with us due to their archetypical themes. Mythic stories have about them the universal elements we can relate to personally.

In heroic myths, the hero, or protagonist, is usually involved in a journey connected with a quest. The hero must move physically from *here* to *there*. The passage is never an easy one. It's usually fraught with danger, demons, dragons, or some such.

But in order for the hero to be the hero (or heroine), the journey must be undertaken. Invariably while making this transcendent journey, the hero becomes stuck, seemingly overwhelmed by horrible, insurmountable barriers and unable to proceed or extricate him or herself in any way. Or, there might be a question to be answered or a riddle or puzzle that he or she must solve.

Anyway, there is always some type of trial involved in the journey. The hero or the heroine must face some type of dilemma, and the situation is never clear.

In myths, when everything seems disastrous, it's crucial that the heroes remain true to themselves, even though they know they may ultimately be defeated. If the heroes hang in there, sticking to their principals and loyalties, a transcendence occurs and invariably something or someone—like Gandalf the Magician—comes to their aid offering a different perspective. This new insight changes everything and provides hope for success.

(This archetypical theme of rescue holds some truth. Sometimes insights and solutions come from surprising places.)

Having faith that an answer exists is a beginning. Staying with the situation and trusting that change is sometimes a painful process allow for new things to emerge.

Consider this: potentially we all have within us the capacity to become the heroes or heroines of our own life histories.

You are the leading actor in the story about a lifelong journey that began at the time of your birth. Naturally, as you travel your life path, you will encounter huge roadblocks, tragedies, challenges, and uncertainties. But you can also discover new meaning and experience triumphs, develop character, and perhaps even gain wisdom.

Life's full of dangers and unplanned circumstances; that's evident. Obviously, you have felt powerless in some situations. It's not really about what happens to you in your life that shapes what you eventually become, but rather how you are *affected* by what has taken place in your life. It's all about what you *thought* about what happened and how you *felt* about it.

It's what you felt and how you reacted inwardly that determined who you are today. There will always be points during your life at which you must make pivotal decisions. These critical decisions are based upon what you know at the time—and they may seem to be the best decisions available.

These choices may not in the long run provide you with the consequences you expected, but these crucial decisions, even if they turn out to be crummy, can always be used as learning opportunities. Try believing that your choices do matter on some important inner level, whether they turn out to be the "correct" ones or not. By pursuing the choices you make, you shape what you will ultimately become. It's up to you to decide whether to grow from this cryptic process or be diminished by it.

But even the present you and where you are now doesn't need to remain immutable and written in stone. The past may be the past, but you do have the power to go back over the events of your life and reinvent and reinterpret them to an extent, by reframing their meaning using a different context.

Remember, memory isn't literal: it's part imagination.

Consider that it is within your power to reimagine your role as the protagonist in your life story. Few, if any of us, grew up in the Brady family. Who really would have wanted to? Some of us grew up in good (or not-too-awful) families, but many children grow up in situations of deprivation, cruelty, and abuse and still grow up and become adults with a capacity for compassion and love. How can this be the case?

Perhaps it's because these children possess some kind of inner myths about themselves. They may have belief systems that shelter them from circumstances they cannot control. Or perhaps they find helpful imaginary companions to whom they can turn for nurturing. Or maybe they dream about how they will eventually escape their predicament or develop strategies that they can use to protect themselves in the meantime.

Little kids are great that way. Small and power-less, subject to the adults who control their lives, certain heroic children are provided sustenance by their wonderful, mythical, magical belief systems. So why can't we do it too?

As an adult you might find it helpful to reenvision your early life and see what comes from it. You might discover what mythic themes you recognize in yourself. Try casting yourself in the role of her-oine or hero. Let other people in your life, past and present, take on the aspects you feel they per-sonify. It isn't necessary to be familiar with Greek or Roman mythology. You don't need to see your-self as Zena the warrior princess, or Cassandra, or Hercules, or Jason with his golden fleece. Story time is for everybody. Hansel and Gretel work just as well.

Cinderella could provide a starting point for your personal myth. You might identify with char-acters like Oliver Twist or Harry Potter. *The Lord of the Rings* or *Watership Down* might give you some ideas, you know?

The Mask

How would you describe yourself? How would you explain your identity? Many thinkers tell us that most people go through their daily lives following routines they developed in order to meet needs and to control a limited amount of resources. It's a set of patterned behaviors designed to foster competition and recognition and to control conditions that feel threatening or intolerable.

Well, now the jig is up! The world has changed, and in changing, it has invited your soul to risk removing the mask forged in childhood. Maybe now is the time to let go and discover the true entity within. That person doesn't need to have a set of survival strategies or patterns of action. That person can smile at the outward persona and those silly illusions and archaic perceptions and understandings.

What fearful freedom! What a chance to listen to who you are! Transformed, the true self experiences a shift in perception. There may be a new understanding that just starting something or making one small change can have unbounded ramifications.

When the inner self is accessed, you may find that you really like yourself! You might find that you are behaving like a new person, astonished that you could ever have seen the world as you used to.

Aware that it cannot control much of anything, rather than resist, the inner self becomes free to see itself as malleable and permeable rather than simply vulnerable. It's open to accepting and exploring new experiences and interpreting events in novel ways. Being present, without being resistant, creates new possibilities for transcendence.

Out of fear, too afraid to question, we cover ourselves with the mask. We are so busy embellishing and caring for our masks that we shudder to think that there may be nothing of substance underneath.

Now we'll find out.

Green Nature

What do grasses, open fields, flowers, and vegetable gardens have to do with staying mentally healthy?

Research supports the notion that living in or near green spaces can improve your mood and reduce the effects of stress.

If you live in a big city where you can't easily access a park, you can bring a bit of nature inside. Green plants not only clean the air, but the oxygen they add to the atmosphere can also work at oxygenating your home. The added oxygen can improve cognition, reduce aggression, and enhance an overall feeling of spiritual well-being.

Research also found that after taking a walk in nature, participants reported lightened feelings of depression, decreased symptoms of anxiety, and an increased memory span.

Spending time in natural places can speed recovery from mental fatigue, help slow down heart rate, and lower blood pressure as well.

Studies have shown that veterans, victims of natural disasters, and other people suffering from PTSD (post-traumatic stress disorder), who participated in nature-based rehabilitation therapies, were better able to deal with their PTSD symptoms and developed more positive mental states.

Even kids with ADHD were better able to focus after a walk in the park, compared with their peers who took a walk in an urban neighborhood.

People in schools with a view of a natural environment outside their windows were found to be more alert and productive than their counterparts who had no view of plant life or other types of natural settings.

Studies also indicated than men and women who exercise in natural environments (especially in the presence of a body of water) found improvement in their self-esteem and greater feelings of hopefulness, relaxation, and general overall satisfaction with life.

No green thumb? Not to worry. Here is a short list of hard-to-kill plants that can help turn your place into a little parkland.

- Pothos (*Epipremnum aureum*)

Nicknamed "Devil Ivy," pothos is tough to kill. It's a great slacker plant. It can thrive in plant-unfriendly areas of your home. Low lighting and limited water don't do them in. Many times, they are variegated, meaning some leaf parts are lighter and some are darker, so it's good plant to add visual interest.

And, if you want another, you can simply take a cutting, place the stem in water until it roots, transplant it to some soil, and voila!

- Snake plant (*Sansevieria trifasciata*)

    Snake plant gets a bad name, but it's actually a sweetie, requiring very little maintenance. It actually *likes* low light and dry soil. Who doesn't like that?

    The plants have straight or wavy leaves and can grow anywhere from six inches to ten feet. Pick one that feels good to you, and put it in a place where you'd like to add a little interest.

- Lucky bamboo (*Dracaena sanderiana*)

    While lucky bamboo can grow in soil, the potted ones are grown in water. (Therefore, you can't kill them by overwatering them, a mistake made by many novice indoor gardeners.) A member of the lily family, lucky bamboo needs repotting infrequently as it is slow to grow. Sounds like a piece of cake.

• Arrowhead plant (*Syngonium podophyllum*)

These tropical plants are fast growing. Although tropical, they can bounce back from gardeners who forget to water them. They vine and they bush. If you don't like the vines, simply snip them off and repot directly in soil and watch while they grow a new little arrowhead.

Have fun!

WHAT WOULD HAPPEN IF...

THE RECENT SITUATION, although upsetting and frightening, has afforded us the opportunity to slow down and experience the stillness and to consider compassion not only for other human beings, but also for our very environment, with all its creatures and plant life.

What would happen if, instead of taking a picture on your smartphone to post on Instagram, you simply sat under your umbrella on a creaky old bench in the park and listened to the raindrops fall, pattering in puddles, nourishing the earth?

What would happen if, instead of jumping out of bed to check your emails upon awakening, you allowed yourself to open your eyes slowly as the Eastern cultures suggest?

What would happen if you allowed yourself to transition slowly from sleep to awareness?

What would happen if you were able to take the time to relish the remnants of the dream images that still floated in your mind during that between time (from sleep to waking) and then dissipated like billowy clouds in the breezy air?

What would happen if you opened your bedroom window to the star-speckled night sky and considered the faint moonlight? What if you listened to the curious sounds of the frogs and clicking cicadas? Perhaps you might hear an owl asking "whoo" was listening.

It is at these times that you see yourself in all your anxiety and fear and in all your exaltation. Usually stuffed away with all the business of the day, these feelings creep into consciousness with a certain clarity.

These feelings long for your understanding and even for your acceptance and love. Know that these are your strengths and points of light. They are guides leading you to be grateful not only for your blessings but for your challenges as well.

These feelings, both positive and negative, offer you profound opportunities to awaken and to grow in wisdom.

CONTINGENCIES

WHAT IF THIS were a world without demons, devils, or gods? The universe would take on a new meaning. What would change for you if you knew that our existence was merely happenstance, random—that the world was not designed for us?

Indeed, perhaps the world was not designed at all!

If our species never appeared at all, or if Neanderthals were the dominant species, the world would be a different place with no homo sapiens.

If we are the stuff of stars, simply tweaked by evolution, how amazing and unique becomes our human existence. How special life becomes.

It's crucial that we cherish it.

To be able to share in the knowledge gleaned by other human beings is almost mystical. In becoming aware that we might contribute a bit to the wisdom that is passed on, we take on an awesome responsibility. This body of knowledge is not just instinct, something we know innately, something we're born with. This learning is a malleable, changing thing.

How contingent is our place in the vastness of the cosmos! How miraculous! A self-aware species on an ordinary little planet orbiting an ordinary star in an ordinary galaxy—it sounds like a fairy tale.

We did not have to be, but we are. What then is our responsibility to ourselves and to others?

There is a certain mystery in all of this. Have what we consider to be our cultural constraints been molded from clay that has no reality? Have we been coerced into following rules from another time, another place, from any number of other people?

What if?

Morning Notes

WHEN YOU WAKE up, wake up gently if you can.

When you're not quite fully awake, write a page or two about anything that comes to mind. Make your notes handwritten and single sided—for your eyes only. Do this as fast as you can. Let your thoughts flow, stream of consciousness style.

You might find that this exercise clears you for the day ahead. It gets rid of the leftover debris standing before you and your day.

Kind of like a prayer, in morning notes we are telling the universe what we need, what we want more of, and what we dislike. We access an inner resource. Many people would shy away from the notion of prayer, but what is a prayer exactly? It's asking God, a Higher Power, a Source, or a Force for what we need. It's intentionality. So, it doesn't matter what name we give it. But it may make a difference if we listen to what it tells us.

Call it intuition or a hunch, the upshot is that guidance does come if we are open to it.

You might pooh-pooh this idea and chalk it up to coincidence. But, as we practice becoming receptive, this guidance may become a relied-upon tool. Although the hints can be subtle, we may be guided in unexpected directions.

Paying attention to the subtle nuances can provide us with a shift in perspective that allows for the integration of new possibilities and my guide us in unexpected directions.

LET YOURSELF BE
(A MEDITATION)

ANY TIME IS a good time for meditation, but it's good to meditate before you eat a big meal. Meditation reduces worry and diminishes anxiety.

Take some time to find a place where you can sit comfortably, with your spine in a neutral position, shoulders relaxed. It's not necessary to sit in *padmasana*, (the lotus position) but do relax. Breathe calmly and deeply. Try for a four count as you breathe in, hold your breath a moment, and then breathe out for a count of four or five. (This may seem awkward at first but with practice will become second nature.)

Choose to be present; choose to pay attention. Become aware of your body simply by noting what your body is touching. Notice your clothing and what you're sitting on. Is anything else touching your body? Is the cat rubbing against your leg, perhaps?

Some people find that closing their eyes helps them to direct their thoughts inward. Become aware of any sensations your body is experiencing. Do you feel heat, cold, itching, or pain? If you are sitting outside, is it breezy, sunny, or noisy? Notice that these sensations are pleasant, neutral, or unpleasant. Notice these things and then let them go.

Continue to breathe deeply and calmly. This is the essential message of mindfulness: pay attention. When we're fully present, the universe informs the heart of our being.

Try to be mindful of any negative feelings in your mind and respond to them with a relaxed, compassionate response. States such as gratitude, patience, and generosity help to soothe your consciousness and aid in clear thinking.

Don't try to discount the fact that frightening things can and certainly do happen. Calm and compassionate responses may not help in situations of imminent danger (where your body just responds and the fight-or-flight response automatically kicks in), but they can go a long way in helping to get you through less grave and dangerous situations.

Reflect that you're not the Lone Ranger, not just some separate being sitting there breathing.

You are not just breathing, but being breathed. You live in an oxygen and carbon dioxide–producing environment. You need all the wonders of the oxygen-producing world's vegetation to support you. You need trees and grass and flowers and ferns and the plankton in the sea to support you—and they need you as well. You are intimately interconnected with the living planet. You are reminded that you are a part of everything. Where does the self begin, and where does it end? You are reminded that you are part of it all, part of the wholeness of life.

TOTEM

MANY NATIVE PEOPLE around the world have long believed that each of us has his or her own totem. Often this totem, or helper spirit, takes the form of a particular animal that has significance and relevance for the individual. This totem can be regarded as an animal that is our magical talisman, teacher and our protector. But we must be open to it. We have to accept not only its strengths but also its shortcomings.

The qualities of our totems have resonance for us.

It's not always easy to discover your totem. And once you do, the answer might surprise you. Answering the following questions may help you discover and adopt yours. It might be helpful to close your eyes and take some cleansing breaths before you begin this exercise.

Of all the animals you can think of, wild or domestic, to which animals are you most attracted?

When you were little, what animals did you think a lot about or collect—dinosaurs or horses maybe? Do you still think about them as an adult?

When you go to the zoo, to which animals are you drawn?

Is there an animal that you've dreamed about with frequency? Were the dreams frightening, funny, comforting, strengthening, or maybe something else?

Did the animals in your dreams possess special powers? Could they foretell the future, for instance? Could they speak or dance?

If you could be any animal, what animal would you be?

When you're out in nature, what animals do you hope to encounter?

If you could have any animal for a pet, even a wild one, what would it be?

When you try to answer these questions, it's probable that you will find that you have more than one answer per question. That's OK, but try to think about only the ones that are really important to you. Be just like a little animal (or a little kid) and follow your instincts!

It's a good bet that your totem animal will be the one you answered yes to the most often.

If that particular animal works for you and *feels* right, you might want to think about that animal's qualities, maybe even do a little research on it, and see what you both might have in common. Don't be surprised if you discover that even traits you may initially consider less than fabulous in your totem buddy have some adaptive functions.

Give them a break! After all, in the wild at least, animals can take care of themselves. They don't have problems with self-esteem. They forage for their food and find their own shelter. They don't worry about the S&P index, and they care for their offspring. They eat what's available and *sleep a lot*—apparently with no big problems, so they don't get stress-related illnesses. And most of the time they get along with others of their species.

They don't start wars either.

They know a lot of things that we don't.

They don't even require clothes. (That eliminates a lot of chores, for sure!)

NAMES FOR A COLLECTIVE OF ANIMALS—JUST FOR FUN

Apes: a shrewdness
Bats: a cauldron
Bears: a sloth
Cats: a pounce
Dogs: a cowardice
Elephants: a parade
Giraffes: a tower
Goats: a tribe
Gorillas: a band
Jaguars: a shadow
Kangaroos: a troop
Leopards: a leap
Lions: a pride
Monkeys: a barrel
Porcupines: a prickle

Rabbits: a colony
Squirrels: a scurry
Tigers: an ambush
Whales: a pod
Wolves: a rout
Doves: a dule
Ducks: a brace
Eagles: a convocation
Hawks: a cast
Larks: an exaltation
Owls: a parliament
Ravens: an unkindness
Sparrows: a host
Swans: a bevy
Turkeys: a rafter

Earth's Academy

WE ALL ENTER this life (as does every living thing) through the miracle of birth. In our case, we are conceived by human beings and delivered into the world through the body of another human being, our mother.

Some people believe that we choose the parents to whom we are born because our soul has determined that it is with this family that our soul's growth and its wisdom will be facilitated the most quickly. We are all born into a lineage, a tribe. Sometimes we join a family brimming with love, but that certainly is not always the case. Nonetheless, it is within this context that we acquire life's learnings. Hopefully, we learn from many sources, not the least among them our experiences.

As we travel our personal path from birth to death, we are enrolled by the cosmos in an individualized earth school. In this school experience is our master teacher.

Our individualized academy of being and learning and changing provides us with life's lessons. These lessons can take many forms and provide many challenges. Some of the things that we learn may be quite mundane; other learnings can touch us deeply and be life transforming.

Our personal earth school provides a custom education, not only for our intellect but for our heart and soul as well. All of it depends on our readiness to accept the lessons presented to us in whatever life circumstances we face.

Throughout the ages people have been presented with different challenges and choices. Clearly, the current circumstances are unique. Never before has there been such a challenge on a global scale.

We are invited to weigh our personal choices with discretion, taking advantage of what we have learned. It may not seem like it, but our personal choices can affect the world socially, ecologically, and politically.

By keeping in mind that our impact on the world might be much greater than we think it is, we are given a responsibility. By becoming more conscientious and considered in our decision-making, we might just maximize the positive effects of our thoughts and actions on others and, ultimately, on the world.

It's Not Just Hooey (Hypnosis)

ONE FINE STRESS-REDUCTION technique is self-hypnosis. Actually, all hypnosis is self-hypnosis. You control how deeply you want to relax and follow the suggestions you may receive. You are in a different, altered state, but you're always in control. As it turns out, when hypnotized you are quite self-aware. It's a very pleasant experience. If you like, you can record this induction for yourself.

I'll close my eyes and begin to relax.

At first, I may be much more aware of some things than I was before.

I hear the sounds that surround me in the room where I sit.

I hear a clock ticking and the heater going on (adjust to fit your circumstances).

I hear the sounds of my voice.

I feel the sensations in my feet and my hands.

Thoughts and certain images float without a care into my mind automatically.

With my eyes closed, it becomes easier and easier to become more and more aware of several things that I might otherwise have ignored or overlooked as I traveled through my busy day:

Feelings,

Thoughts,

Sensations.

And now I allow my awareness to become a bit altered; my mind begins to explore and experience a little relaxation, and it lets go of cares and hassles.

I even let go of the effort it takes to be reminded of where exactly my feet are positioned or where my hands hang or how I'm holding my fingers. I let go of the effort it takes to be aware of which leg feels heavier or more relaxed as well.

It seems like it's just too much effort to be bothered with right now.

I will take a moment to experience the letting go, but in my own time and in my own way, even more than before.

I will begin to drift and become more relaxed. I'll let go, and my mind will flow down

Toward a peaceful, simple place

Where there is comfort and safety—

A place where I will remain comfortably aware of what I need to be aware of,

Not worrying, just observing.

This is a place that directs me downward into complete peace and relaxation.

The meaning of my words may almost not seem worth the effort of deciphering.

It's so much easier

To simply relax

And wait,

And allow events to occur almost by themselves.

It's a drifting downward and a settling.

Then drifting back into time and upward toward wakefulness.

And that is just fine too.

It all belongs to me anyway.

I have a conscious mind and an unconscious mind as well.

My mind will continue to hear and understand what is important for me to know.

In my own time and in my own way

I will learn.

My experience will be altered.

I will receive what I need.

My unconscious mind will explore and guide my very awareness as I explore my capacities and abilities.

An Old Friend

Who is this companion of yours? Seemingly such a strong creature, yet neither flesh nor blood with no body and no bones? Neither younger nor older than when he first appeared on the scene. Not born, just there, experiencing all, calmly knowing. Confidently knowing all is well where he is—no one can touch this companion, no matter what's happening now.

This being is never sick; he is always calm and observant, dancing backward and forward with ease and grace—accepting pain and pleasure as all the same, never seen, never heard. Your companion can be maddeningly unreliable; frequently not coming when really needed.

Your companion can gladden your heart or make you feel remorse; bringing you gifts and then taking them back, with no apologies either. He likes to have things his own way. He can frustrate you and anger you, but he can soothe you too.

You'll never change him, but you might be able to see him in a different light. You must treat him with gentle love and forgiveness though, and open your soul to him and all he is. With wisdom, you might find a soft spot in your heart for him, even with all his idiosyncrasies. What would you do without him?

After all, he is *your* memory...

Impermanence

Thinking about change leads us to feel differently about what we consider reality. When we are mindful of this impermanence, we pay more attention to change in ways we may already be aware of but take for granted or overlook.

There are the obvious changes we experience with nature, such as day and night, the seasons, or even broader things like climate change. On an even larger scale, we know about evolution and the rise and fall of various civilizations. We know flowers bloom and then decay. We know people are born and then die.

Considering that we have all these examples and a myriad more facing us every day, it's astonishing that we still find changes in our lives surprising and sometimes unsettling.

When we are mindful, we see that new things

come and old things go. Things arise and disappear.

We are among the few generations that will witness the grand finale of the world as we have known it. We are, as author Jean Houston calls us, "the people of the parentheses." We live at the terminus of one era, but haven't quite reached the new one.

As an exercise in mindfulness, it can be helpful to notice what part of change predominates for us. Do we see new things arising, or do we see endings more clearly; or do we see both? Does it matter if we consider the coming of change to be a good thing? Or has the going away been of more benefit to us?

Neither perspective is right or wrong. It's just something of which we can become aware.

The Whole World
Smiles with You

It's true what your grandma told you: smiling is good for you.

Your brain knows when you are smiling and decides to throw a party. This releases little molecules called neuropeptides that help fight off stress. Then other neuropeptides come to the party—serotonin, an antidepressant, does a little polka with its friends the endorphins, the pain-relieving neuropeptides. Everybody feels good!

Smiling can reduce the heart rate and boost your happiness level. Authentic laughter does the same. If you don't believe it, you may want to fake a smile and see what happens. When we smile, people tend to smile back. It's like yawning; we can't help it and react with a smile. It's a little happiness loop, and it can feel pretty good.

As Thich Nhat Hanh says, "Sometimes your joy is the source of your smile, but sometimes your smile can be the source of your smile."

In the workplace, smiling and laughter can affect your job performance. Researchers have demonstrated that happiness has a positive causal effect on productivity. It can make you a more efficient and creative worker.

Laughter is the definition of healthy. —Doris Lessing

CAT'S CRADLE

MANY PEOPLE, IN many different cultures, believe in the idea of reincarnation. They believe we have several chances at living and that if we don't do it right the first time, we will have subsequent opportunities to learn all we need to. In other words, there are many lessons to be learned from living and from varied opportunities, and as part of the meaning and mystery of life, it's our mission to try to learn them. Different cultures and religions have different methodologies for accomplishing this learning. That's not really relevant for our purposes, and it doesn't matter if you go along with this belief system. It only matters that you play along for right now.

What if you knew you'd have, say, eight chances to be reincarnated? So, you have a chance to learn and evolve through nine lifespans. You'd basically be the same person, but you would have different things to assimilate over the course of maybe four hundred years or so. What if you even had a choice in deciding what type of things would interest you or what types of lives you would like to live? Would what happened in 2020 change all that?

If you didn't have only one life to live—and you knew it—would you attempt different things? Like a cat with nine lives, would you lead one life that was simple and spiritual, one that was adventurous, or one that was sensuous? Would you devote one lifetime to helping others or to intellectual pursuits, or live one life that was physically strenuous? Are any of these incarnations extremely attractive to you? Do some appear disagreeable but necessary in order to learn to achieve what you must?

What do you think your ultimate quest would be? What goal would you like to attain to give your existence meaning?

Make a mental note of the types of choices you might make. As you pass through your day, take a mindful minute to notice all the things that take place. See if any apply to the different scenarios you considered.

How might you apply any of these learnings in your present incarnation?

PERSONIFICATION

ONE DICTIONARY DEFINES "personification" as the attribution of human nature to inanimate objects or abstract notions. Poets do it all the time with concepts such as loyalty, love, and honor. Probably, though, to one extent or another, all of us tend to adopt certain concepts, feelings, and moods and ultimately identify them with ourselves. If you had to think about a personified concept and whether or not it applied to you, could you? Below is a list of items to consider. Try not to choose the one you like the best. For instance, don't choose blue because it's your favorite color. Try to discover what word best *defines* you and makes you the most *knowable*.

Tumultuous changes have taken place that have rocked our concept of self and our sense of self-efficacy. Perhaps you'll find that you are thinking about yourself in novel ways.

If you had to decide, which color would best define you in your present mood? Have you always been that color?

Which number resonates for you? Has that changed?

If you had to choose one, which element—earth, wind, fire, or water—shares qualities with you? Is this a new you? Have you always had qualities of that element?

If you were a flower, what type of flower would you be?

What season do you associate with yourself? Is this a temporary thing, a new thing?

If you had a special time of day that resonated with you, what time would it be? Are you always comfortable with that time or does your time change with the seasons or your health, or for some other reason? Why?

Do you see all these associations as positive or somewhat negative? Do they make you feel happy, melancholy, blessed, spiritual, competent, mercurial, or inspired?

Do you see them as positive strong points or negative weaknesses? In what ways do the personifications you own affect your sense of who you are?

As you pass through your day, notice how perceived associations affect your behavior or your mood. Try using this framework as you observe others.

Can you use this system when thinking about your partner, spouse, parent, or child?

Does this framework supply you with any insights concerning the fashion in which these individuals operate?

Does it change how you might feel about or interact with them?

Can this new understanding help you to better empathize with them?

Smoke and Mirrors

Have you ever considered this? Every action, everything we do, is based upon some belief we have about what's going on. We're just acting on assumptions really. Our whole life, our whole way of feeling about ourselves, is based on guesses or on things somebody taught us about the way life is and how things work. What? You say, I know that this or that is the way things are. I know that so-and-so is true! Do you? Sometimes truth can be just as subjective as reality.

As you place your fingers on your computer's keyboard, you assume something. You bet that the computer screen will register the word you type and the computer's hard drive will save every little word for you. This assumption is rather implicit. You don't, after all, consciously think about whether or not the computer will work each time you sit down in front of it, but it seems like it probably will be based on your experience. Usually these types of cause-and-effect assumptions are pretty reliable. The notion seems to be empirically correct at any rate.

It's not necessarily always the case though, right? All our knowledge is experiential after all.

What about the assumptions you make that have some type of emotional impact on you? If you believe someone enjoys your company or thinks you're witty and wonderful, or conversely if someone ignores you or is cruel to you, you'll likely base your behavior on those assumptions. Those assumptions, however, might not be at all scientific or provable, and they're certainly not necessarily correct.

How could reality be so fragile? How could we base everything we do on assumptions or acts of faith? And many of these acts of faith are implicit. We don't even know they are just assumptions. *We never question them at all!* It's important to think about this. Such beliefs may control how we feel about our relevance and efficacy in the world.

Moreover, unfounded beliefs can cause us to see ourselves as saints or sinners, brilliant or banal, and not one whit of it might be true. Since they remain unexamined, these possibly unfounded lifelong hypotheses hold us prisoners to certain consequent behavior patterns. These behavioral outcomes may not have any relevance to reality at all. Our assumptions can make us miserable or elated, depending on the emotional baggage they carry, and they may be thoroughly off base. They are founded only on our unexamined prejudices and belief systems.

What are some of your beliefs about life? Have you tested them lately?

Consider that, in life, situations are not easily definable as black or white and that we are clearly attached in an emotional fashion to many of our beliefs. In fact these beliefs can put a slant on our entire life. They can distort our perceptions and cause not only happiness but also a lot of grief and pain.

Values

So many of us have plenty, and yet somehow we remain dissatisfied. We are more materially comfortable and secure than our ancestors could have ever dreamed of being. Our twenty-first-century society has offered us the values of materialism, individualism, science, and rationalism and provided us with more safety than several other peoples around the world; still many people are not satisfied or fulfilled. Perhaps that's because all the material comforts have carried with them the precariousness of our present situation. It could all be lost. It could all be taken away.

COVID has taught us that. So, then what will we have? We are vulnerable to loss through sickness, want, and death. Besides that, many people in our society have come to feel displaced. People feel lost, alone, and empty.

Maybe the feeling of lack lies in the fact that few of us take time to nourish the nonwork aspects of our lives. Maybe things are out of balance. Could it be that when we search for ways to grow other aspects of ourselves, we will become healthier and more fulfilled? It can be lonely living with just your intellect to run things.

What about the spirit part of humans? Not spirit in the limited sense of vitality, but rather in the sense of energy that goes beyond our normal, everyday, bringing-home-the-bacon, material selves.

Is the spirit just a fantasy, just a delusion?

What about love? Is love simply a matter of pheromones, just a biological imperative for preservation of the species, or is love a form of transpersonal energy as the mystics believe?

What about intuition? Is it just an instance of a great hunch as a rational person would confirm? Or does intuition come from some deeper place? Is it truly a special kind of knowing?

And compassion? Is compassion only a display of some do-gooder trying to get points, or is it a genuine concern one being has for another and the recognition that we are all, at some level, brothers and sisters?

Then there are mystical experiences, those precious moments when time seems to stop and everything feels in sync. Psychologists call such episodes of congruence aha moments when we are in the "flow." Are these intense and benevolent encounters with oneness an instance of genuine transcendence or merely the dream of a small, lonely creature who fears dying?

Maybe we can't come up with answers to these kinds of questions, but perhaps they are worth considering. If we're nothing more than material bodies, cosmic-chemical anomalies/accidents, we may as well go for all the material gratification we can get while we can. If, on the other hand, we are more, it seems likely that the more deeply we explore our spiritual side, the richer we will become.

THE WEB OF CONNECTION

WE PERHAPS PERCEIVE the web that is the world the most clearly, and the most real, when we fracture it a bit. We follow the fissure with a baleful eye. The ruined part will need some repair. The connections stand out once they've been severed. We see the connections that bind our lives to all others.

Just as different seeds pursue different paths to germinate and grow, just as they require different conditions and different signals to sprout, we recognize how all things are interrelated. Our lives follow similar patterns. Although not soil chemistry, there are some things we need in order to flourish; that is to say, we need our own special *terroirs*. Our needs make these things no less urgent and necessary.

A beaver meddles and builds a dam on a river. There are implications. The current is affected.

Organisms and insects cluster; birds perch and leave their droppings. New plants begin to grow.

As participants in society, there is no way that our actions won't have some effect on the world. Each and every decision we make—from the way we behave toward animals and toward other human beings, to the things we eat, to the organizations we belong to, to the ideas we espouse—has some influence in some way on those around us. We can't predict the effect our beings and our plans will set in motion.

Simply watch and wait and trust that things are as they should be.

Allow the web to enfold you in its embrace.

TIME TRIPPING

Do YOU EVER allow yourself to be transported back in time to the world of childhood, where everything was clear and fresh and full of wonder? Can you visualize a time before you had everything classified, before the very words and names that could enhance your experience had also taken things away? Before your perception was programmed? It sometimes seems that once we label things, we stop bothering to really look at them or see them.

Step outside some starry night. Settle in. Go to a place out there and in there where concepts and labels no longer obscure what you experience. Allow the subtle intimations of your higher truths and higher knowledge to explore. Look and see. What do you feel? What do you know? Can there be any real knowing without wonder? Can there be any real knowing that is not embedded in the sense of the sacred out there and inside you?

You probably know it's all a game. It's all made up. This success and failure thing. You have to decide who's going to make up the rules. Or you can decide to invent your own. We have come to a place where we must invent a new game whose rules are largely unknown. The past may not prevent or predict the future, and in the new game you might also want to throw out other pesky things like measurements of success and failure in value judgments. You could even get rid of comparisons and competition and base the whole deal on new stuff entirely. In the new game, concerns like how you measure up and how much you make and where you rate your social standing could all be chucked! It doesn't mean that such items are unimportant or frivolous. It just means that the old stuff, the old models of behavior, carry with them limitations for being, and that may not work in the New World. Is your life about the same things now as it was, say, twenty years ago?

Sometimes new games can provide you with paradigm shifts in the way you look at life and allow for alternatives and new ways in which to solve problems, if only briefly. They may even allow for new ways of solving problems. New games can whisk us away from some of the grimmer facts of everyday reality.

Every contribution you make affects the world, although you may not have the slightest inkling of how.

WHAT THE WORLD MEANS NOW

HAVE YOU EVER really thought about what the world means to you? Do you feel as though you have a connection to it, or do you feel you are alienated in some ways? Do you value it only in so far as it can gratify your needs?

What is that tree outside your window; is it humanity's trust or simply some fuel for the fireplace? And mountains, are they mainly sources for timber and other resources or do their peaks hold a deeper significance?"

We once heard in song that we were "stardust," we were "golden." Does that concept resonate in your present life? Maybe more than maudlin sentimentality, perhaps the human soul continues to yearn for continuity in connection and companionship with the world. (COVID has certainly taught us that we are all connected.)

It might be that an enhanced sense of communion with the natural world can help us to become more mentally healthy and to live more ethically and more genuinely, and can supply us with a sense of the sacred that seems to have been snatched from the modern world.

Maybe traditional societies know something that we "moderns" have forgotten. Ethical codes can be explained by their concerns with encompassing all of nature. In those societies, plants and animals and rivers and mountains took on a certain spiritual significance and were honored in their own way.

If we reject the sacredness of the world, how can we believe in the sacredness of humanity?

Are our hopes of immortality only wistful dreams?

INNER WISDOM

MANY PEOPLE SEEK someone to look up to, someone who can act as their guru or their role model, hoping their teacher's insights will help to guide them on their life's path. In fact, finding the right person to mentor you is fine. However, relying on your own wisdom is equally, if not more, valuable. You are gifted from birth with an innate wisdom that cannot be learned and can lead you on a path to self-realization.

We don't have to travel far to find our bliss. Joy is a built-in aspect of our inner self. As you travel on your path to personal transformation and learn more about yourself, you'll gain in self-discernment.

Discernment is a human wonder power! It's our internal guidance system that comes from the very core of our being. It's our ability to know what's right. Sadly, we have been trained not to trust our inner wisdom. We may look outside ourselves for saviors to save us from our predicaments. We look to rituals, though we rarely get them quite right. We rely on saints and heroes to guide us through the quagmires of our lives.

But our inner wisdom isn't dependent on the outside world. The world can't persuade us to act in opposition to our values. We retain our free will.

Wisdom is the source of discernment. No other force you encounter will contribute as much to your capacity to do what is necessary to be who you want to be.

So, if you're on your path and looking for some guidance, turn to yourself. The right answer may not be obvious, but if you ask and let go and wait, your answers will come. And on your path, you'll find the way to your true potential,

What's the Point?

What's the point? Maybe it's just about being happy. If this is so, we must still find the definition for happiness. Perhaps happiness doesn't really have much to do with things like honor or wealth or pleasure—things that you want or feel you have to have.

Maybe happiness is more of an action verb. It might just be about remaining consciously aware of your human capacity to actively and continually do the best you can to be happy. Perhaps it's about living, working, and relating with a purpose and seeing ourselves within the larger context of our humanity. When we live life outside the context of our connection with other people, we miss out.

It seems that if we can connect our own interest to something bigger than ourselves, we grow spiritually. By incorporating a heightened sense of community and an appreciation of our environment, perhaps we can provide ourselves with an enhanced perspective on true happiness. Life flows when we turn our attention to larger patterns of which we are all a part. Life sparkles with new meaning when we can transcend the imperatives of our personal survival.

Many of us long for a way to extricate ourselves from who we've been or who we appear to be. But how do you make the transition? After all, you've played a role for so long, and you played your role so convincingly. It's what others expect of you, is it not? How can you find a way to break free of old patterns that might have functioned pretty well but no longer fit? Now that everything's upended and in transition, what will become of you without known parameters for living? There is no way of escaping it. Well-worn patterns are outgrown and need to come apart; we begin to question assumptions that once seemed right. The truth no longer seems so simple. Patterns have brought us to where we feel more like tight, rusty shackles than helpful guides. We must, it seems, become like olden-day explorers charting unknown territories and crossing unknown seas in hopes of finally reaching new destinations. In order to do this, one must be something of a romantic. You have to genuinely be in love with people, places, and adventure because there will surely be times when you feel terribly lost and need to find value in wherever you chance to be and in whomever you chance to meet along the way.

THE SMUGGLER

A MIDDLE EASTERN FOLK TALE
ATTRIBUTED TO MULLAH NASRUDDIN

A CLEVER SMUGGLER came to the border with a donkey. The donkey's back was heavily laden with straw. The official at the border was suspicious and pulled apart the man's bundles until straw was all over the place, but not a valuable thing in the straw was found. "But I'm certain," said the official, "that you're smuggling something!"

The man was nevertheless allowed to cross the border.

Each day for ten years the man came to the border with a donkey piled high with straw. Although the official searched and searched the straw bundles on the donkey's back, there was never anything to be found. He could find nothing of value hidden in them.

Many, many years later, after the official had retired, he happened to meet the same smuggler in the marketplace. The smuggler was dressed in fine robes, finer than anything the official could have afforded. He had clearly grown quite wealthy.

The official said, "Please tell me, I beg of you, tell me what you were smuggling. I know you were smuggling something. Tell me what if you can."

The man looked down and smiled to himself. "Donkeys," he said.

Sometimes, what you're looking for is right there in front of you, if you're not too busy with your own beliefs to notice.

You May Just Need
a Pep Talk

THERE ARE TIMES we all feel uncertain about our capacity to accomplish what we are trying to do and to overcome the challenges we must to reach our goals. Sometimes we may feel as though we are just plain incapable. One way of overcoming doubt about our capabilities is by replacing this negative self-talk with more positive and inspiring affirmations.

Bring to mind your negative beliefs about your abilities and eventually replace them with statements in which you affirm your talents. Think about other times when you have succeeded in gaining what you wanted, and remind yourself that the challenges at that time seemed insurmountable, but you did succeed, and you do have the capacity to succeed again.

This may initially be difficult to do; it may feel phony. But you'll find that if you stick with it, eventually you'll begin to own these affirmations and empower yourself to go after your goals with an increased feeling of purposeful mastery. Your negative beliefs will disappear.

It's easy to forget that we do have control of our self-limiting thoughts and unproductive self-talk. We can turn them around, making us feel more adept and proactive concerning our goals.

In doing so, a new level of competence and mastery can be achieved.

HAIKU

I love to haiku
Could be you might like it too
It's simple to do

THE REAPER

So, what about illness, what about death?

The world's main spiritual and religious traditions address these subjects in their own ways, promising hope for salvation, another chance, an end to life's suffering, or the hope of nirvana among them.

Doubtless, though, many of us accept the temporary condition of our incarnation as everything. We accept this life as our endgame, our permanent truth, when we accept our mortal, physical selves as our true selves.

No wonder then that when we think in such a fashion, we see our illnesses as problematic, no doubt as monstrous calamities. Perhaps we try to isolate ourselves in an abundance of material things in order to divert our attention from the, perhaps, unbearable fact that ultimately, we all die.

The illusion is that perhaps we can live forever. We hang success and fame and money like magic bangles in front of our eyes in vain attempts to forestall the inevitable. No one is exempt. We all leave the material world, and no amount of money, science, success, fame, or prayer will change that fact.

It is this illusion, this very ignorance of the true situation, that blocks us from being comforted by the consideration of our full reunion with the universal oneness of everything of which we are all a part. We are all equal in the face of death, yet we abhor the grief a bit, although along with grief there may come some measure of compassion and love.

There are unfortunate people who have never had the luxurious chance to think about these things. Death takes them too early or by surprise. Others are luckier and have the opportunity to gaze upon the door as it slowly opens and consider what their life has meant in the scheme of things.

Enough (A Meditation)

WE ACT ACCORDING to how we feel not how we think. One way to work with how we feel, even with negative feelings, is to welcome them into our meditation. When we sit with our feelings, even the unpleasant ones, we can make friends with them. Rather than trying to develop strategies for escaping, minimizing, or avoiding our negative feelings, befriending them offers us another option and allows us accept the wisdom they have to offer.

First, take a few deep breaths (can you feel your breath coming from your abdomen?). Scan your body and turn your attention to the negative emotion you're feeling to see where it's living in your body. Can you determine whether it's in your shoulders, your neck, your back, your heart, or perhaps your head or your face? Does it feel heavy or constricted, or does it feel like something else entirely?

Let the attention you pay to it be gentle like a Good Samaritan who comes along when you need some companionship. (This visitor does not label it and is nonjudgmental.) You may even welcome your feeling. We spend so much time suppressing, shutting down, or trying to escape negative feelings; notice how this gentle acceptance affects your negative feeling. Sit with it and see what happens next; stay open. It is just a feeling that wants to be noticed and considered. Let it teach you what it will.

If you make a habit of this practice, the feeling will no longer be a threat to you. It will begin to feel safe, relaxed, and liberated. Dwell with it without effort.

It is enough.

POWER TRIPPING

HOW EASILY DO we allow ourselves to be seduced by the concept of power, either our power over others or conversely their power over us? How much of it is simply illusory? How many fewer negative implications might it have if we just became more aware of its shenanigans?

When you think about it, having power means many different things and takes many different forms. The doctrine of *might makes right* has obvious historical significance. Certainly, power comes to us under several guises—some legitimate and helpful, others not so legitimate.

What is your relationship to power? Could you forgo using it? How subtle are you in utilizing the power that you do possess? How profoundly would you have to change if you relinquished your powerful stance over others, if you allowed yourself to value others equally? Power can be a double-edged sword used to help and inform, or it can be used coercively. How do we make the best use of our power?

It might be useful to examine the ways in which power operates in your life.

Referent power is legitimate and refers to the power a person possesses due to his or her personal characteristics, such as charm, charisma, and affability. If you're lucky enough to have characteristics like these, you likely have a modicum of personal appeal and referent power. Hopefully, you use charisma in a positive way and not with coercive motives.

Another type of legitimate power derives from a person's position. You may have this type of power due to your role as a manager, boss, supervisor, or parent.

Power as an expert may be yours if you have a specialized type of knowledge, expertise, or talent in a certain area. Teachers and doctors fall in this category. Again, this type of power is great as long as it's not used negatively.

Another type of power is derived from a person's ability to give benefits or rewards to another. Power like this is benign as long as it's not used to control others.

A fifth type of power, coercive power, is the

type used to control and punish another. This punitive power tripping is the one to guard against in your personal repertoire and to be on the lookout for in other people's behavior.

As you interact with other people, become aware of how the give-and-take of power, yours as well as theirs, affects your moods and behaviors.

Epiphany

ARE THERE MOMENTS in your life that stand out as glowing, as numinous? Can you recall brief states of perfect luminescence, when time stood still and everything just *felt right*? Were there ever occasions when everything else, all the little circumstances of the day, grayed to obscurity, and only these brief snippets of time had relevance, had radiance? Were there ever times when your breath seemed to stop and you dissolved into oneness with your experience?

If you're lucky, there have been times as an adult when you've experienced such states. If not, maybe there were times in your childhood that felt like this. As adults, it sometimes seems people ignore or discount such feelings. Sadly, many seem to lose the capacity to experience them altogether. Perhaps, if we can become more conscious of the mysteries in the small delights of the world that surround us, we can more easily access these times of wonderful harmony and wholeness.

THE INNER CRITIC

WE ALL HAVE one to some extent. Walt Disney cast Jiminy Cricket in the role. Some people call it a conscience, but there is quite a difference. Psychologists use the term *inner critic* when they talk about that little voice inside you. This voice can frequently be a trickster as well. It doesn't only help you to figure out what's right and what's wrong. It tells you about what's wrong with you too.

At first, it seems as though the voice is trying to protect you with its warnings about your vulnerabilities. Then, after a while, it throws in a few cracks about your inadequacies and shortcomings. Does this critic speak the truth? Maybe, but in many cases this critic, who was born in your childhood and brought up right next to you, is just an echo of lessons learned back then that may not be accurate at all.

Before you react to its messages take a moment to listen carefully. How does it speak and what does it really tell you? What appears at first to be a caring protector can become a harsh destroyer as it whittles away at your self-confidence, self-worth and creativity. The critic is only too happy to make comparisons and judgment calls comparing you to others and pointing out that you don't measure up to some sort of nebulous standards that may not apply to you at all.

It's easy to fall into the hands of the critic if we forget to challenge it. If we don't take an active stance and talk back to the critic we have no choice but to listen. It's hard to acknowledge the good things about us and the good things that happen in our lives when we are overcome by the critic. Be gentle with yourself.

Shoulds

We all have "shoulds." They're based on our age, our culture, our socioeconomic group, any number of things. These are the internalized rules that by which we operate. They're the family rules that get passed down from generation to generation.

In some families the rules can be pretty far out, but the kids assume everybody does things the way their family does. They don't get any reality checks. There may be no way for them to explore alternate behavioral rules, so the family rules remain intact.

Many of these internalized rules that you learned in your childhood may come to mind. Cognitive psychologist Albert Ellis called these parental edicts shoulds.

These rules may not necessarily be bad. Societies do, after all, need some kind of a consensus about the way things should be done and what behaviors are acceptable and what behaviors are not, So that's OK as far as it goes. Keeping your shoulds operational is fine as long as they aren't causing you pain or problems in your life or your relationships.

What someone considers to be little differences can mean a lot sometimes, such as when partners disagree and neither is willing to compromise.

As an adult, you can make an assessment of the shoulds that continue to operate in your life. Do they really make sense? Are they still valid? Are they still working for you?

If not, a behavioral update may be needed.

SQUASHED FEELINGS

MANY PEOPLE ARE not at all in touch with their emotions. We've been taught, at least when we are around people, to politely restrain from enumerating our "unacceptable" beliefs and feelings. When asked how they are doing, people usually throw out the canned response, "Oh, I'm doing just fine. How about you?"

Well, maybe that's a safe answer, but maybe it has rubbed off on us even in private, nullifying our actual feelings. These disconnects can cause stress and inflammation as we guard against being aware of our true state of being and honoring it.

Decades of mind-body researchers have suggested that there is no demarcation zone between feelings and the body. What our mind and emotions know, the body manifests. It's known that people who suppress their emotions, as well as those who become volatile in expressing them, increase their risk of stress-related illness and heart disease.

Our "monkey mind" distracts us with crazy-making negative self-talk. That mind is critical and judgmental and can overcome us with worry. We need to become more consciously aware, more mindful, of how instantaneously our thoughts grasp at us. As French author René Daumal tells us, we must "beware of the surface of things." Much of this negativity is simply not worth worrying about.

Take a piece of paper and fold it in half. On one side, list all the things in your life that provide you with energy. These items could include being around certain people, wearing a certain outfit, taking walks in nature, or snuggling with your dog. On the other side, list things that zap your energy or what makes you crazy or angry.

After you've created your lists, turn over your piece of paper and write down a few ideas about how you can let go of some of the things that steal your energy. And how can you increase the things that are energy boosters?

Becoming more aware of these items may steal the thunder from the energy thieves and may empower you to find ways to become more energized and less inflamed.

Hit your personal reset button and provide

yourself with unstructured time—simply listen to some music, paint a picture, play solitaire, or tickle the cat. You could even take a nap; whatever floats your boat!

Connect with your inner child to replenish that which the burnt-out adult has put aside.

Be compassionate with yourself; you'll feel better for it.

THE RULES FOR
BEING HUMAN

AS YOU REMEMBER to give other people, as well as yourself, the benefit of the doubt, and when you can admit that it's not actually within your power to be absolutely perfect, you can begin to let down your guard and find a little peace. As you become more forgiving of yourself and others, you'll find that even little things can make you happy if you just take note of them.

Hopefully this collection of musings and meditations will encourage you to look at your life in new ways. Possibly you'll make some changes that enhance your feelings about yourself and others. Revisit it any time you want to refresh your purpose.

Consider these ideas:

- You will receive a body. You may like it or you may hate it, but it will be yours for the entire period of this time around.
- You will learn lessons. You are enrolled in a full-time informational school called life. Each day in this school you will have the opportunity to learn lessons. You may like the lessons, or you may think of them as irrelevant or stupid.
- There are no mistakes, only lessons. Growth is a process of trial and error, experimentation. The "failed" experiments are as much a part of the process as the experiment that ultimately "works."
- A lesson is repeated until it is learned. A lesson will be presented to you in various forms until you have it down. When you have learned it, you can go on to the next lesson.
- Learning lessons does not end. There is no part of life that does not contain lessons. If you are alive, there are lessons to be learned.
- There is no better place than here. When your "there" has become a "here," you'll simply obtain another "there" that will again look better than "here."
- Others are merely mirrors of you. You cannot love or hate something about another

person unless it reflects something you love or hate about yourself.

- What you make of your life is up to you. You have all the tools and resources you need. What you do with them is up to you. The choice is up to you.

Your answers lie inside you. The answers to life's questions lie inside you. All you need to do is look, listen, and trust.

You will forget all this. You can remember it whenever you want.

—Anonymous

FURTHER READING

Benson, Herbert, and Eileen M. Stuart. *The Wellness Book*. Secaucus, NJ: Birch Lane Press, 1992.

Gawain, Shakti. *Creative Visualization*. Berkeley, CA: Whatever Publications, 1978.

Harp, David. *Three Minute Meditator*. New York: MJF Books, 1999.

Knaster, Mirka. *Discovering the Body's Wisdom*. New York: Bantam, 1996.

Spreads, Carol. *Breathing: The Abc's*. New York: Harper and Row, 1978.

Wells, Valerie. *The Joy of Visualization: 75 Creative Ways to Enhance Your Life*. San Francisco: Chronicle Books, 1990.

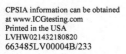